What Do Babies Eat?

How to Lose Adult Weight with the Baby Food Diet

By: Richard Parker

9781635014884

PUBLISHERS NOTES

Disclaimer – Speedy Publishing LLC

This publication is intended to provide helpful and informative material. It is not intended to diagnose, treat, cure, or prevent any health problem or condition, nor is intended to replace the advice of a physician. No action should be taken solely on the contents of this book. Always consult your physician or qualified health-care professional on any matters regarding your health and before adopting any suggestions in this book or drawing inferences from it.

The author and publisher specifically disclaim all responsibility for any liability, loss or risk, personal or otherwise, which is incurred as a consequence, directly or indirectly, from the use or application of any contents of this book.

Any and all product names referenced within this book are the trademarks of their respective owners. None of these owners have sponsored, authorized, endorsed, or approved this book.

Always read all information provided by the manufacturers' product labels before using their products. The author and publisher are not responsible for claims made by manufacturers.

This book was originally printed before 2014. This is an adapted reprint by Speedy Publishing LLC with newly updated content designed to help readers with much more accurate and timely information and data.

Speedy Publishing LLC

40 E Main Street, Newark, Delaware, 19711

Contact Us: 1-888-248-4521

Website: http://www.speedypublishing.co

REPRINTED Paperback Edition: 9781635014884:

Manufactured in the United States of America

DEDICATION

This book is dedicated to Jeanne – who stood up for me when the world seems to be my enemy. Thank you for keeping sane for both of us.

TABLE OF CONTENTS

Chapter 1 - Should You Go On a Diet?

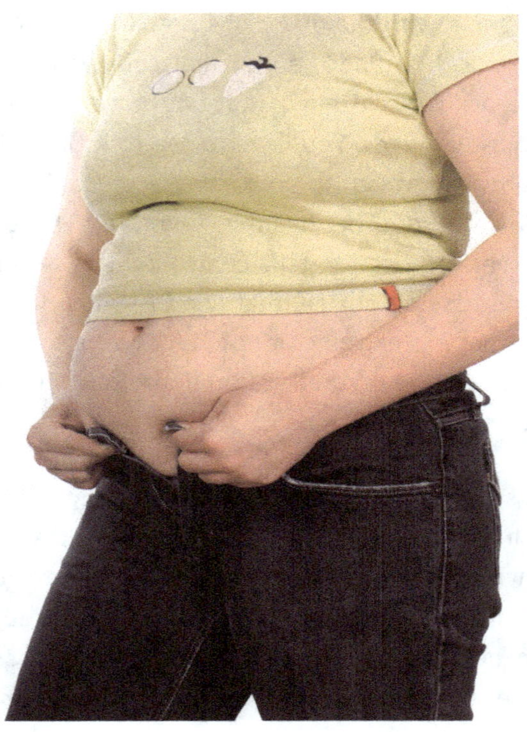

There are a lot of reasons why people want to lose weight. It varies from health reasons to fad or just because you are too pressured with looking good so that people will like you. No matter what reason you have in your mind, we all comes to a common denominator of getting the body we want for our own benefit and happiness. Since there are a lot of hopefuls of losing weight in an instant, there are also a lot of diets coming out.

However, not all diet plans work out just the way it has been promoted. But this does not mean that the diet is fraud, it's just that it doesn't suit you at all. It's just like paper is to pen, when paper and pen are used together best results would come in a form of writing or drawing. But when you paired paper with water, it will just be ruined or you would pair paper with another paper, nothing will surely happen.

It's just the same with the diet plans prepared before you; all you need to do is to first find the diet that suits your body and your need. There are certain things that you have to consider before pursuing your diet plans. You have to see to it that you know how much weight you need to lose. You just can't let things be overdone; it will not be healthy anymore. There are certain limitations that you need to take control of. It is very important as well that you assess your general health status. In every activity you do, whether it is extreme or not, it may be a simple procedure, your health should be secured first and foremost. If there is a need to consult an expert then so be it.

You should see to it that your body is prepared for all the transition that could happen to you. You know for a fact that with the diet plans you will be taking, there are adjustments to be made and your body will be the first part to comply with this adjustments. It would then be fair that you take a thorough assessment before anything else would follow. Furthermore, it will be important that you have the right attitude for this.

Often times, many diet plans would fail not because it is not effective but because of the poor attitudes users put into it. They only give few chances for the diet to work, you should remember that stages are to be taken by your body, and it doesn't mean that because you have started this diet plan today then you'll get fit the next morning. It will definitely take some time and you have to wait for it with joy and satisfaction. You should also know that discipline is one of the most important keys that you should consider.

It is a fact that there will be thousands and millions of temptations that will come your way as you try to get fit. You shouldn't be lame in fighting them. It should keep you still with your goal of getting fit. After all you can't afford to fool yourself, bear in mind that you are deciding for your health and the moment you do something bad, it will be you who will suffer most. More importantly, it will be best that you take note of the things that you like and don't like. This way, things will be put in place just as you wish.

There is no need to punish yourself by depriving yourself with all the things you love. It will only cause you a lot of stress and disappointments. It will not be a joyful journey for you then. It will also be great if you take into consideration your fitness level because this will determine on how you should take action on your losing weight plans.

How Many Calories Do You Really Need Per Day?

There are a few things that determine how many calories a person needs in order to maintain a healthy body. The number of calories that you should consume depends on your age, gender, height, and weight. The number of calories that a person needs to consume on a daily basis varies from person to person. Other factors need to be taken in to consideration while determining as well such as your level of daily activity. It is important that when you determine your number of allowed calories that you are sure that the calories you have consumed will be burned off during the day.

There are several things to consider when designing a diet to limit calorie consumption. One of the most important is your level of activity. You do not want to deprive yourself of needed nutrients but at the same time you do not want to flood your body with calories that you cannot burn off. The best way to avoid this is do some basic math.

What Do Babies Eat?

You must first figure out how many calories you currently burn per day. There are calculators on many health websites that are designed to help you with this process and make it much easier for you. Once you have determined how many calories you burn a day you begin the rest of the process of setting your calorie intake guidelines.

The next step is to figure out how many calories you need to consume regarding your current weight. If you are larger you need to consume fewer calories. Calories can easily turn into fat if not burned off during the day.so that is why it is important to limit them, especially if you are above average weight. At the same time, you cannot cut down your calorie intake too much because this will not have positive results.

If you are burning more than you are consuming your body will begin to burn muscle instead of fat. This is because fat cells serve as emergency reserves for your body so your body naturally tries to burn that last if it thinks it is malnourished.

After you have determined how many calories you need with your weight for your diet it is time to add in the age factor. Most adults need fewer calories than they did in their younger years. This is because older adults are much less active than they were in their earlier years which lead to less calories being burned. As stated before, you do not want calories being left unburned in your body, they turn to fat. So if you are younger and active you will likely need to consume more calories but if you are older and less active less calories is the way to go.

Gender:

It is believed that men seem to need more calories on a day to day basis than women. This is due to the fact that men and women's bodies are different. We have different muscle structures from each other and therefore our bodies burn different amount of calories on a daily basis.

For example, an active male can require more than 3,000 calories a day when they are active. This means that they engage in sports or other activities which cause the body to work. The recommended intake for the average woman is 2,160 calories per day for an active woman. That is quite a big difference, isn't it?

Height:

This is pretty much common sense. If you are taller you are going to need more calories due to the fact that you have more body mass than shorter people. The more of you there is the more calories you need. Always remember, eating too many calories will lead to a gain in weight and setbacks in your diet. If you are trying to create a more healthy body and life for yourself then over indulging on calories is the last thing you want to do.

I hope that these tips on calorie consumption have been useful for you and have answered some of your questions. Keep in mind; diets need to be personalized to an individual's needs so what another person needs in calories will likely be different than you needs.

Trying to copy somebody else's diet because it works for them will likely have negative results for you since you will not be getting the balanced diet you need. There are also websites that have calorie calculators and these can help you greatly while you are trying to determine your number of needed daily calories.

Chapter 2- Defining the Baby Food Diet

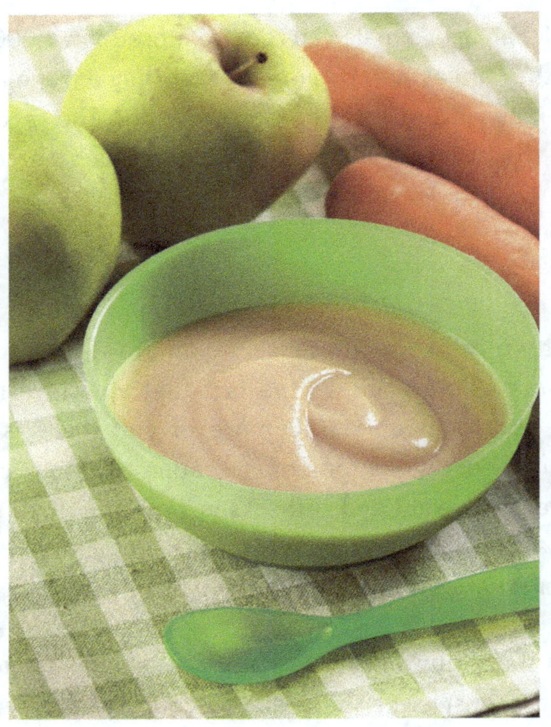

There are a lot of diet plans that we can acquire, it may affect us in so many ways but the fact will always remain that we would want to try all the means to be fit. One of the new trends that have been around is the baby food diet. It is actually formulated by Tracy Anderson. She is known to be the trainer of the celebrities which allows them to attain the body they have now.

It is true that such diet is a fad but whatever it is, it all comes down to a point of allowing you to lose weight. That is the most important thing that you will get the body you've always wanted. And because this is created by a celebrity trainer we can then be assured of the fact that it is made with utmost care. After all this will be used by public figures and they can't just adopt to any diet plan. They have to see to it that they are getting the best of the best.

The diet plan is actually made through a pureed baby food which makes sure that all low caloric content will be utilized. Thus, you have to be very meticulous that you are getting the right components and the right ingredients, if you miss on these then chances are it won't work just as you planned it to be. It will take some time though to be sure that you get the right thing done. However, you shouldn't be afraid because you can look into guides all over the internet.

It is true that it has spread worldwide through internet and it will not be that hard for you to get a list of this. All you need to do is to do your own little way of research and everything sets into place just the way you wanted it. One more thing about the baby food diet is you will be helped as you try to discipline yourself. Have you ever thought on how will it help you discipline? Well, baby foods are usually stored in a small jar and because of this you can be assured that the food you will be taking is enough to maintain the discipline. Through this, you can be sure that there will be a small amount taken every meal as you follow the baby food diet. This is actually one of the common problems all dieters are facing; it will be hard to take control of the amount you will be eating.

If you would avail of the baby food diet, you can make use of the small jars just to see to it that you will be that religious to follow your diet plans. It is important that you will be aware as well that this baby food diet is not at all limited to every meal; you can actually take this as a snack which can be taken in between the meals. Thus, you will be assured that you are taking a healthy diet and you can continue getting this as your daily meal. You can absolutely feel good as you are getting the body you have but you are not at all sacrificing the nutrition your body needs.

What Do Babies Eat?

One good thing about this is you are not at all obliged to follow specific rules unlike other diet plans. It will be all up to you on how you plan to consume your baby food diet. You can actually follow on your regular meal and have your baby food diet as a snack. Some would opt to take baby food diet as a regular meal. The truth is there is no specific exercise routine required when you follow baby food diet. However, it will always be best if you take your baby food diet with proper exercise not just to trim down but to get fit and healthy.

Why is Baby Food a Trending Diet Plan?

Have you ever thought that one day baby food would be one of the most trending diet plans? Well, it is a fact that in the past baby food is used to feed babies alone. After all it consists of all major nutrients and you can be assured that it is all nutritious. You should know that it will be a total package since it would be given to growing children which foremost need the best diet they could ever have.

In the end, it has been thought that because of the many people suffering from unhealthy weight and we just can't let go of the fact that its number is increasing from time to time. Therefore, something has to be down to eradicate this present situation. The food experts then find a way to help those suffering from excessive weight to lose weight without sacrificing their nutrition need. Without too many sufferings you will be able to reduce your weight in no time and you can be assured that you will really lose weight the healthy way.

It is true that having an excessive weight will lead you to a lot of problems. It is not limited to just being unable to follow the trend but it will make you suffer a lot of illnesses. You can actually get high blood pressure and heart attack in lined with your weight.

Thus, it will be better if you take your weight seriously for as long as you can. You should know that your health is one of the most important things that you have to consider because having a good health will allow you to live a happy life. You can then do things that you love and enjoy most. It is true that baby food diet is new to us and some of us may find it hard to believe in this craze but it does work. You will definitely lose kilograms without getting unhealthy.

The fact is you will actually get healthier than the usual diet plan because with this diet, you will not be forbidden to eat the food you love. Furthermore, the diet is quite known thus we can say that it is true to its word and it thus makes you healthier and sexier. Despite that, you should be aware of the reality that this will not work if you don't get the exact amount of calories. That is why it will be best that you take good control of your needs. You shouldn't take things for granted when it comes to your food intake because it will surely get into your nerves of you take it loosely. You should know that getting this diet will not be that hard because what you need is to stick to a 14-jar baby food diet each and every day.

It is a fact that this diet will help you get a sumptuous dinner without crossing your diet plans. You can still go on with your diet just as you planned it as you take baby food diet in your hands. More to that, it will be best if you have an idea of how this baby food diet is made. This will be the time then that you can say how healthy your diet is. It is made out of mashed bananas, pureed veggies and even meat.

When you look at the ingredients, you can definitely say that you are getting a complete meal. With this kind of diet, you will be able to get your body used to certain kind of diets thus you will slowly decrease the calories in your body. In the end, you will realize that you have patiently waited until good results will come.

"It's Not a Crash Diet Plan"

Despite the fact that you are on diet, you still receive the same amount of nutrient that you need each and every day. However, you should be aware though that the baby food diet is equated as a crash diet plan because if you get to have one or two baby food diet per day, there is a chance that your calories will suddenly drop. If you have this you might actually find it hard to adjust and make your body be aware of the change that would come.

Just be sure that when you are in diet, it doesn't matter what kind of diet you are in for as long as you are into it, it will be best that you never starve yourself and deprive with all the good things in life because it will not help you get the weight you desire. It is definitely unhealthy to keep on getting this kind of result. It will be better if we get healthy as we practice healthy living.

As with baby food diet you can be sure that you will get the best result because it has a complete ingredient that is all set for your need. You will have the chance to get hold of a jar of baby food as a snack or even a meal. You can be assured that with this kind of intake, you will be able to get the best of everything just as you need it. You can be sure that you will be healthy all the way. Despite the fact that you are on diet, you still receive the same amount of nutrient that you need each and every day. However, you should be aware though that the baby food diet is equated as a crash diet plan because if you get to have one or two baby food diet per day, there is a chance that your calories will suddenly drop. Thus, it only add up to your stress which could hinder the weight lose you are cooking for. Thus, it only add up to your stress which could hinder the weight lose you are cooking for.

Richard Parker

There are actually a lot of flavors when it comes to baby food diet and it will be all up to you then on which diet you prefer most. Just keep in mind that whatever flavor you choose it will leave you with the same effect and that is it will make you fit at the healthiest possible way you can imagine. In lined with this, there is a chance that you will definitely feel weak. You will feel weak not because you are not getting the exact nutrient needed but because of the sudden change of caloric intake.

It is important that you'll be aware of the fact that you need to take your diet one step at a time. Furthermore, the pureed baby food diet that is placed in small jars will allow you to get the discipline you truly need to reduce over eating. It will no longer be that hard for you to control your food intake because of the fact that you will be given in jarred meal.

It is important as well that you will be aware of the fact that there are a lot of advantages that you will get aside from keeping a controlled diet because it contains measured diet plan that is all set on giving you a nutritious meal that will definitely help you achieve your desired body in no time. However, you have to keep in mind that there is still a need for you to control eating baby food because you might actually over eat and that will not be of benefit to you then. According to the experts only few adults get to tolerate this kind of diet and it will only take few weeks before you would stop eating it.

CHAPTER 3- SHOULD YOU GO VEGAN WITH THE BABY FOOD DIET?

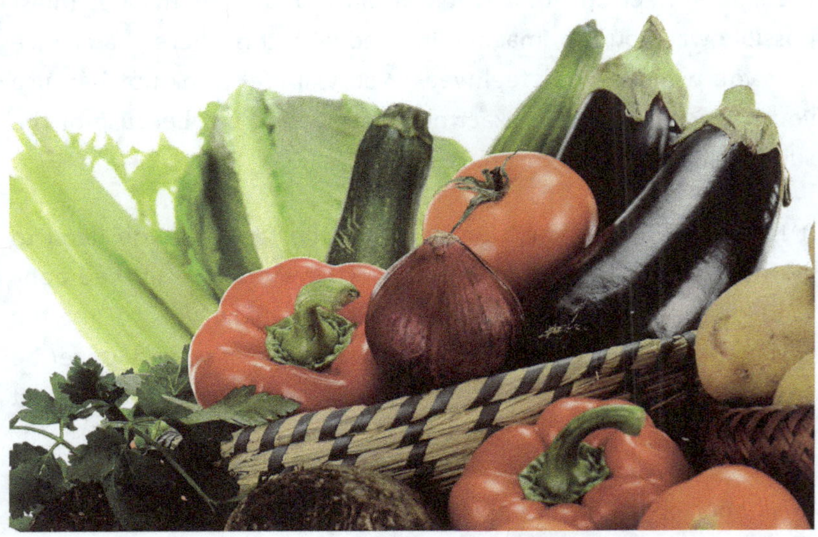

Being a vegetarian is already healthy but it will be healthier if you get it with baby food diet. It is definitely healthier of you choose vegetarian baby food diet. If you are a vegetarian and you want to take your diet to another level then this will be the best choice for you.

It is a fact that as a vegan, you will get to adjust to any kinds of diet that easily because your body is quiet used to the portions of intake you are having each and every day. Before anything else it will be important that you will be aware of the fact on how vegetarian diet works. When we say vegetarian, they are actually having a meal that is out of meat. That is why you can say that it will not be hard for them to take good control of this kind of diet because they are all used to eating a meatless food. It is important that you will be aware that you take these two diets at one so that you will definitely get the full effect of it. If you would combine it, it will definitely be a blast on your end.

It is important that you'll be aware of the fact that when you are a vegetarian your diet is not balanced since you are depriving yourself of the other things you need. You are not even eating meat that is required for a complete meal. Often time's vegetarians suffer from deficiency of the following: calcium, iron, riboflavin, zinc and even Vitamin B12. When you look at all of this, you would actually think twice if you would really want your health to suffer as much. You might actually start asking on why is this so, now that you are eating vegetables you would definitely look at it as a healthy diet plan but the thing is there are certain components that are not available with veggies alone. You would definitely want to have meat in your diet still but in minimal amount. However, with the new diet found in town you can definitely have both sides of the world. You can use the baby food diet so that you will be healthy without sacrificing anything.

There are actually certain recipes that you could follow so that you can be sure of the proper diet you need. You can actually start with carrot and lentil puree. All you need is a cup of peeled and diced carrot; you will also need a cup of dry lentils with small onion chopped together with a tablespoon of olive oil and four cups of water. After you have gathered the ingredients, you can now start heating your sauce pan and sauté it with onion. You will then add lentils and carrots.

The next thing that you will do is to pour in water until it will reach boiling point. You can then cover the pan until it will simmer. Be sure that you will be able to soften the lentils and let in cool before you would have it pureed. The next recipe that you could take is the pumpkin and barley dinner. You don't have to worry actually of it will be very easy to make. You will have to chop the pumpkins and have it soaked in s drained barley. You will now then put one and a half tablespoon of olive oil, the small onion and crushed garlic. You will also need 3 cups of vegetable stock and some thyme and sage leaves. You will then cook all of the ingredients but you have to make sure that you will have it pureed.

A Proper Diet is a Balanced Diet

You need to have a diet consisting of well-balanced healthy foods and not a bunch of junk food garbage. The saying goes "you are what you eat" so therefore if you eat a bunch of crap food you are going to feel like crap. The same goes for healthy food. If you consume healthy foods on a regular basis as part of a healthy diet you will surely feel great and not have to deal with the side effects that unhealthy eating cause.

If you are a person who has not felt quite like themselves for some time now and are not sure what is going on with your body, have you ever considered that it may be your diet? The food you consume determines the health of your body. If you constantly eat junk food your body will likely be in a low state of health. It will be easier for you to get sick and fight of illnesses; you will feel sick, low on energy, and sometimes even irritable. These are normal side effects of a poor diet. It only makes sense as our body needs certain nutrients to be able to function properly. If you rob your body of these essential nutrients it will do what it has to in order to make sure it makes it so see another day. In many cases, the body will cause undesirable side effects to itself in order to try to give you a hint that you need to start eating better.

Dieting can also be very beneficial for people facing certain mental strains in their current life. A proper diet can be very beneficial for the mental health of a person. Just like the rest of the human body, the brain needs certain essential nutrients in order to function properly. Not consuming a proper diet you will likely become easily stressed or overwhelmed as your brain will be deprived of the nutrients it needs to function.

Richard Parker

It is your body and you only get one so you really need to take care of it. You need to remember that your body should be thought of as a temple and not a place that should be filled with bad things. Only let the best things in your body and keep the bad stuff away. I know this is easier said than done but with effort and determination it is possible.

CHAPTER 4- THE TRUTHS BEHIND THE BABY FOOD DIET

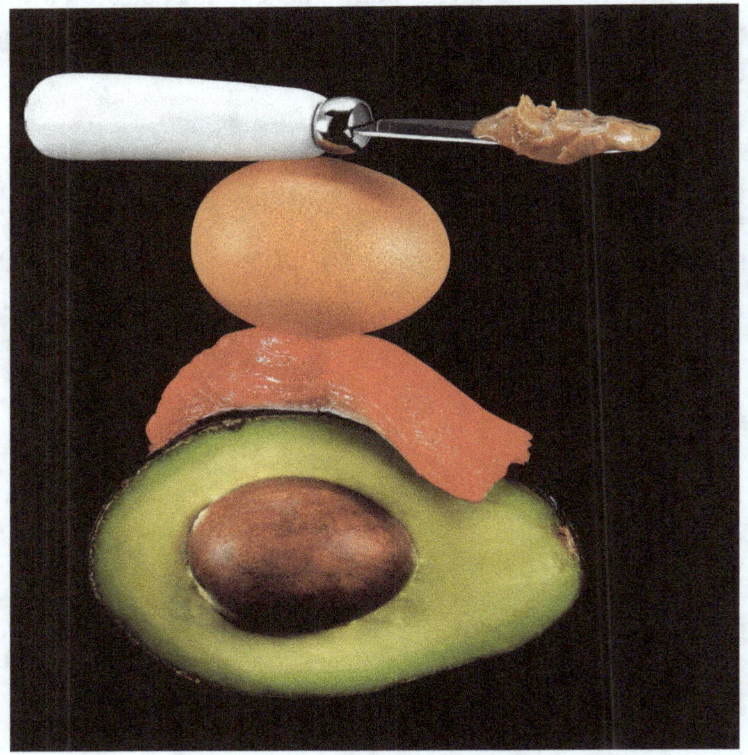

It's just the same with the diet plans prepared before you; all you need to do is to first find the diet that suits your body and your need. There are certain things that you have to consider before pursuing your diet plans. You have to see to it that you know how much weight you need to lose. You just can't let things be overdone; it will not be healthy anymore. There are certain limitations that you need to take control of.

It is very important as well that you assess your general health status. It will definitely take some time and you have to wait for it with joy and satisfaction. You should also know that discipline is one of the most important keys that you should consider. It is a fact that there will be thousands and millions of temptations that will come your way as you try to get fit. You shouldn't be lame in fighting them. It should keep you still with your goal of getting fit.

After all you can't afford to fool yourself, bear in mind that you are deciding for your health and the moment you do something bad, it will be you who will suffer most. It is true that such diet is a fad but whatever it is, it all comes down to a point of allowing you to lose weight. That is the most important thing that you will get the body you've always wanted. And because this is created by a celebrity trainer we can then be assured of the fact that it is made with utmost care. After all this will be used by public figures and they can't just adopt to any diet plan. They have to see to it that they are getting the best of the best.

The diet plan is actually made through a pureed baby food which makes sure that all low caloric content will be utilized. Thus, you have to be very meticulous that you are getting the right components and the right ingredients, if you miss on these then chances are it won't work just as you planned it to be. More importantly, it will be best that you take note of the things that you like and don't like. This way, things will be put in place just as you wish.

There is no need to punish yourself by depriving yourself with all the things you love. It will only cause you a lot of stress and disappointments. In every activity you do, whether it is extreme or not, it may be a simple procedure, your health should be secured first and foremost. If there is a need to consult an expert then so be it. You should see to it that your body is prepared for all the transition that could happen to you. You know for a fact that with the diet plans you will be taking, there are adjustments to be made and your body will be the first part to comply with this adjustments. This is actually one of the common problems all dieters are facing; it will be hard to take control of the amount you will be eating.

If you would avail of the baby food diet, you can make use of the small jars just to see to it that you will be that religious to follow your diet plans. It is important that you will be aware as well that this baby food diet is not at all limited to every meal; you can actually take this as a snack which can be taken in between the meals. Thus, you will be assured that you are taking a healthy diet and you can continue getting this as your daily meal.

The Proper Meal Portions

You should know that it will be a total package since it would be given to growing children which foremost need the best diet they could ever have. In the end, it has been thought that because of the many people suffering from unhealthy weight and we just can't let go of the fact that its number is increasing from time to time. Therefore, something has to be down to eradicate this present situation. You can then do things that you love and enjoy most.

It is true that baby food diet is new to us and some of us may find it hard to believe in this craze but it does work. You will definitely lose kilograms without getting unhealthy. The fact is you will actually get healthier than the usual diet plan because with this diet, you will not be forbidden to eat the food you love. Furthermore, the diet is quite known thus we can say that it is true to its word and it thus makes you healthier and sexier. Despite that, you should be aware of the reality that this will not work if you don't get the exact amount of calories. This will be the time then that you can say how healthy your diet is. It is made out of mashed bananas, pureed veggies and even meat.

Richard Parker

When you look at the ingredients, you can definitely say that you are getting a complete meal. With this kind of diet, you will be able to get your body used to certain kind of diets thus you will slowly decrease the calories in your body. In the end, you will realize that you have patiently waited until good results will come. That is why it will be best that you take good control of your needs. You shouldn't take things for granted when it comes to your food intake because it will surely get into your nerves of you take it loosely. The food experts then find a way to help those suffering from excessive weight to lose weight without sacrificing their nutrition need. Without too many sufferings you will be able to reduce your weight in no time and you can be assured that you will really lose weight the healthy way. It is true that having an excessive weight will lead you to a lot of problems. That is why you can say that it will not be hard for them to take good control of this kind of diet because they are all used to eating a meatless food. .

You might actually start asking on why is this so, now that you are eating vegetables you would definitely look at it as a healthy diet plan but the thing is there are certain components that are not available with veggies alone. You would definitely want to have meat in your diet still but in minimal amount. However, with the new diet found in town you can definitely have both sides of the world. You can use the baby food diet so that you will be healthy without sacrificing anything.

It is important that you be aware that you need to take these two diet plans at one in order to get the full effect of the diet plans. If you would combine it, it will definitely be a blast on your end. It is important that you'll be aware of the fact that when you are a vegetarian your diet is not balanced since you are depriving yourself of the other things you need. You are not even eating meat that is required for a complete meal.

What Do Babies Eat?
Is the Baby Food Diet Enough to Keep You Energized?

There are actually a lot of diet plans that are spread worldwide yet it is fact that there are a lot of crash diets that are never losing its trend. It is true that many of us are still using a lot of crash diet even if the fact will always remain that it has a lot of unhealthy effects, not only to our health but more importantly to us as a person. It is definitely unhealthy to keep on getting this kind of result. It will be better if we get healthy as we practice healthy living.

As with baby food diet you can be sure that you will get the best result because it has a complete ingredient that is all set for your need. You will have the chance to get hold of a jar of baby food as a snack or even a meal. You can be assured that with this kind of intake, you will be able to get the best of everything just as you need it. You can be sure that you will be healthy all the way. Despite the fact that you are on diet, you still receive the same amount of nutrient that you need each and every day. However, you should be aware though that the baby food diet is equated as a crash diet plan because if you get to have one or two baby food diet per day, there is a chance that your calories will suddenly drop.

If you have this you might actually find it hard to adjust and make your body be aware of the change that would come. In line with this, there is a chance that you will definitely feel weak. You will feel weak not because you are not getting the exact nutrient needed but because of the sudden change of caloric intake. It is important that you'll be aware of the fact that you need to take your diet one step at a time. Never ever try to rush things out because it will definitely harm your body in general and this is not healthy anymore. It is a fact that with crash diets, you will definitely feel weak because you will not be satisfied with the food intake you are getting. If you think that it will still be hard for you to take the baby food diet alone then it will be best that you take regular meals in between.

You can also incorporate unsweetened granola or bran so that you will not totally starve. Just be sure that when you are in diet, it doesn't matter what kind of diet you are in for as long as you are into it, it will be best that you never starve yourself and deprive with all the good things in life because it will not help you get the weight you desire. Thus, it only add up to your stress which could hinder the weight lose you are cooking for. There are actually a lot of flavors when it comes to baby food diet and it will be all up to you then on which diet you prefer most.

Just keep in mind that whatever flavor you choose it will leave you with the same effect and that is it will make you fit at the healthiest possible way you can imagine.

CHAPTER 5- BABY DIET FOOD RECIPES

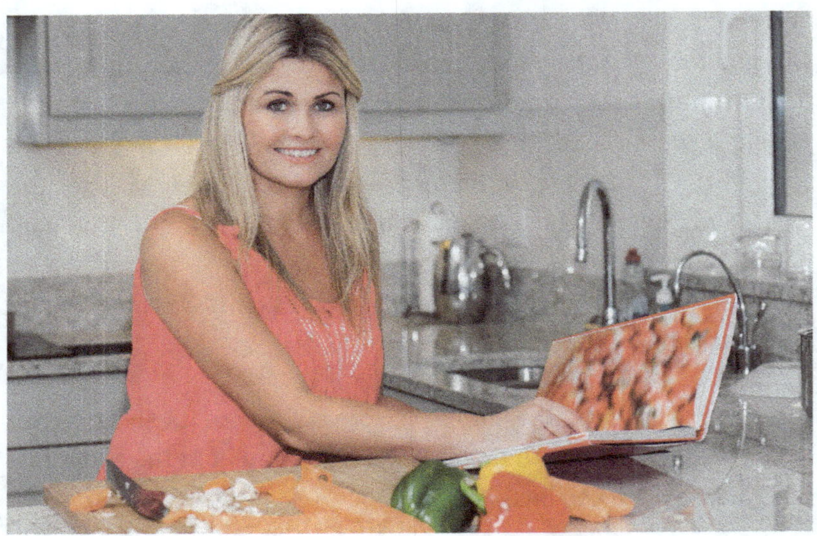

It is a fact that there are a lot of things that we have to consider when it comes to choosing the right diet that we deserve to have. One of the many concerns of those seriously taking into account the fact whether they would take on the baby food diet or not is not having enough nutrition from the baby foods they will be taking in for quite some time. Well, we couldn't move away the fact that things have to be taken into consideration because it will affect your health status the most. Having that at hand is totally unacceptable and baseless.

The baby food diet is considered as one of the healthiest diet programs that we could all enjoy. The foods that you will be eating when you are into the diet are basically the same with the normal dietary plans. The difference would be it will come in a different package. It is true that there are many healthy baby food recipes that are made to provide complete nutrition for all individuals who seeks for a healthy way to make them fit. You should know that the smaller servings provided for you as a daily intake then you will definitely be helped as you foresee an effective control on excessively eating.

It is a fact that everybody will be in unison in saying that all baby foods are healthy because first and foremost they are part of the community that needs to be taken very carefully. After all, many parents would rather trust the baby food they provide for it to be eaten by their infants. They have to be sure that the food they provide will be enough to feed and nourish babies. You should be aware that jarred baby foods has different flavors, texture and food types and it will be all up to you on which you prefer most. You can actually check the labels for their nutritional contents so that you can definitely choose the right diet that you perfectly need.

It is important that you will be aware of the fact that there are those who prefer cooking their own baby foods; it will not actually matter if you choose to have it this way for as long as you make it sure that you're cooking all the good ingredients and not just any other food that couldn't contribute to a healthy diet at all.

The baby food you will be cooking should comprise vegetables, fruits, beans, whole grains and some lean meat because this are the ingredients that will make it a healthy food diet. Furthermore, it will be best that you should avoid taking in sugars, fatty meat and buttery ingredients because that will definitely not make good of you. There are actually a lot of food diets that you can consider doing when you are at home.

Below are few of the many baby food recipes that you could look into.

TURKEY DELIGHT

Ingredients:

Pound of ground turkey meat

A rib of celery,

A small onion

A small carrot,

A can of cannellini beans

Fresh sage leaf

One tablespoon olive oil

Two cups chicken stock

Procedure:

The first thing that you should do is to wash and peel and dice the onion, celery and carrots into small pieces. In a medium stock pot, you can start heating oil and sauté the turkey until it browned. Be sure that you will remove the turkey and set aside for later use.

The next thing that you can do is to add the celery, onion and carrot dice to the same pot and cook for around seven minutes. With that you can now add back the turkey and mix well. Then you can now add the stock, beans and the sage leaf. Be sure as well that you cover and bring the pot to boil. Once it is boiling, you can now turn down the heat and let simmer for another 10-15 minutes.

Let it cool then for a while. Once the pot is completely cooled, you can now use a blender or food processor to puree the food cooked.

It is important that you'll be aware of the fact that turkey meat provides relevant amount of protein, choline, phosphorous and selenium, while beans are rich in calcium, magnesium, copper, Vitamin A and zinc.

LAMB AND APPLE DINNER

Ingredients:

A cup of minced or ground lamb

One medium apple, grated

One zucchini

One medium carrot

Half cup of apple juice

Pinch of cinnamon and tarragon.

Procedure:

The first thing that you could do is to heat it low so that you can slowly cook the lamb in a medium pot. You can use the fatty juices for further cooking. When the meat is almost done, you can now add the carrot, apple and zucchini bits and pour in the apple juice. Be sure to stir it properly so that you can mix it well and cover the pot. Let it simmer for about 15 minutes then before you would add the spices and continue cooking for another five minutes.

What Do Babies Eat?
Now all you'll need to do is to cool it completely before mashing or pureeing the mixture.

Your Own Little Way of Research is Required

All you need to do is to do your own little way of research and everything sets into place just the way you wanted it. Through this, you can be sure that there will be a small amount taken every meal as you follow the baby food diet. You can absolutely feel good as you are getting the body you have but you are not at all sacrificing the nutrition your body needs.

It is a fact that this diet will help you get a sumptuous dinner without crossing your diet plans. You can still go on with your diet just as you planned it as you take baby food diet in your hands. More to that, it will be best if you have an idea of how this baby food diet is made. This will be the time then that you can say how healthy your diet is. It is made out of mashed bananas, pureed veggies and even meat.

When you look at the ingredients, you can definitely say that you are getting a complete meal. With this kind of diet, you will be able to get your body used to certain kind of diets thus you will slowly decrease the calories in your body.

One good thing about this is you are not at all obliged to follow specific rules unlike other diet plans. It will be all up to you on how you plan to consume your baby food diet. You can actually follow on your regular meal and have your baby food diet as a snack. Some would opt to take baby food diet as a regular meal.

It is true that many of us are still using a lot of crash diet even if the fact will always remain that it has a lot of unhealthy effects, not only to our health but more importantly to us as a person. It is definitely unhealthy to keep on getting this kind of result. It will be better if we get healthy as we practice healthy living.

As with baby food diet you can be sure that you will get the best result because it has a complete ingredient that is all set for your need. You will have the chance to get hold of a jar of baby food as a snack or even a meal. The truth is there is no specific exercise routine required when you follow baby food diet. It will not be a joyful journey for you then. However, not all diet plans work out just the way it has been promoted. But this does not mean that the diet is fraud, it's just that it doesn't suit you at all.

Using the Principles of Baby Food Diet to Lose Weight

The baby food diet has been a hot Hollywood diet craze which comes from small jars of baby food which allows you to take small amount of food based on the container alone. There are a lot of people starting to eat three to four jars of baby food on top of their regular meals. They see to it that despite this new set of diet, they get to eat regular meals that are often eaten regularly at equal portions. You should really see to it that you will be eating enough regular meal because depending on the baby food alone will not be enough especially in your first few tries.

You need to support it with regular meals so that you can stand your fight with losing weight. But if you would insists on using the jars for regular meals then be sure that you get enough meal especially when you are replacing more than just a snack. You should know that with every little jar, it only consist of 200 calories. That is why it will be very important that you will learn what your needed calorie is so that you can compensate well. On a lighter note, you have to consider the benefits and the advantages you will be having as you utilize baby food diet.

What Do Babies Eat?
On the practical side, baby food is placed in a small jar which does not require refrigeration. You can simply store it at any storage box, for as long as it will be safe then it will definitely be fine and will all be ready for you to be eaten in time. More to that, your choices on the different kind of food will not be limited, you definitely have a lot of choices. There are a lot of flavors that you could choose from and it will be less of a hassle on your end because there is no need for you to cook the baby food once it will be placed in the jar. When you feel like eating it now then you surely can and more to that you can carry it anywhere you would want to go.

The most important thing is that every baby food is placed with vitamins and minerals that will make it healthier. You will definitely be given the chance as well to have a measured meal that will be enough to control your eating habits. However, you should always remember that in every good thing we encounter there are negative parts that you can consider. You should know that there are no medical instructions packed along with this baby food diet plan thus you will get best results from this.

And more importantly, the baby food diet has no evident taste compared to the ordinary food. It is important that you'll be aware of the fact that there are no sugars, salt and any other seasoning added on this specific diet. Therefore, you should expect a not so tasteful food. Furthermore, since this is pureed you will feel a mushy texture as you will eat it. Therefore, you can say that this may not satisfy you the most but it will content you with the nutritional aspect of life. All you need to remember is you should also take your part so that your diet plan will work.

CHAPTER 6- THE PROS AND CONS OF THE BABY FOOD DIET

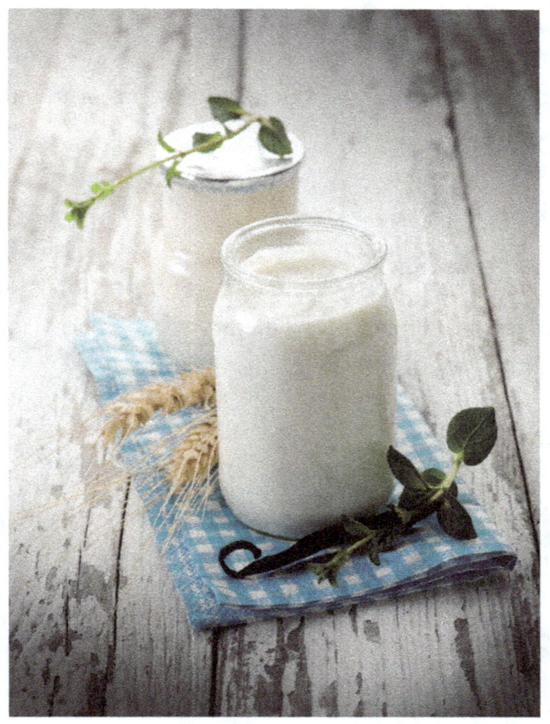

In everything we do, there will always be good and bad side and you have to face it with all your heart. You should see to it that you will take things at hand so that you will have a better understanding on what you are going through. You shouldn't allow other people to control your views about the said baby food diet. This will only happen if you get to have hands on experience about this.

It is very important that you will take things very seriously when it comes to this since you are talking about your health and this is not just something that you could forget about and move on. From time to time, you will see the effect it will have for you if you don't take things passionately.

What Do Babies Eat?
The Pros

1. It is made out of fruits and vegetables

Baby food diet are usually made out of fruits and vegetables which is usually pureed thus you will be assured that you will be getting enough vitamins and minerals.

2. Intake Discipline

It is very obvious that you will have a good portion of your intake because the food is placed on small jars and it is now separated for you. All you have to do is to follow it religiously.

3. Additive-free

Since this is a baby food, you can be assured that it will not be added with various chemicals that will not be good for your health at all.

4. Ease Your Cravings

It is a fact that this will ease your cravings because this could replace your snack requirement. You can definitely have this for snacks.

The Cons

1. Cost

It is a fact that baby foods are quite expensive because of the very meticulous way of having it.

True enough, it will make you feel tired if you would continually eat the same food over and over again. Despite the fact that there are a lot of flavors available, you would still find it mushy to eat the same food over and over again.

A Few Reminders when Following the Baby Food Diet Plan

It may be because of the fad of having beautiful body that van be flaunted to nay public event. However, it is hard for most of us to find the right diet that could fit our need. It is important though that we take dietary rules at hand because we may find it hard to adjust on the different kinds of diet present before us. It has been said that the amount of baby food you will be consuming every day will differ depending on what is your daily calorie goal, it will also matter on how much weight you wanted to lose and how fast would you want to get to the bottom of this.

On the other hand, it is important that you'll be aware that the baby food diet has diversity as well that you have to consider. There are actually a lot of ways that you have to look into because of the different methods that would replace the complete meal you should have taken all throughout the day. That is why it will be very important that you will learn what your needed calorie is so that you can compensate well.

On a lighter note, you have to consider the benefits and the advantages you will be having as you utilize baby food diet. On the practical side, baby food is placed in a small jar which does not require refrigeration. You can simply store it at any storage box, for as long as it will be safe then it will definitely be fine and will all be ready for you to be eaten in time. More to that, your choices on the different kind of food will not be limited, you definitely have a lot of choices.

There are a lot of flavors that you could choose from and it will be less of a hassle on your end because there is no need for you to cook the baby food once it will be placed in the jar. However, come would consider using the baby food as a snack replacement because most of the snacks would be too sweet and it will just ruin your wish of getting your body according to how you wish it.

The baby food diet actually works by decreasing you caloric intake without sacrificing your nutritional intake. Good thing that baby food diet comes into picture because it will allow us to get fit without actually sacrificing our health. Before anything else comes to existence, it is important that we dwell on the past so that we will all have a better idea on how this baby food diet started.

Chapter 7- Diet and Exercise Should Always Go Together

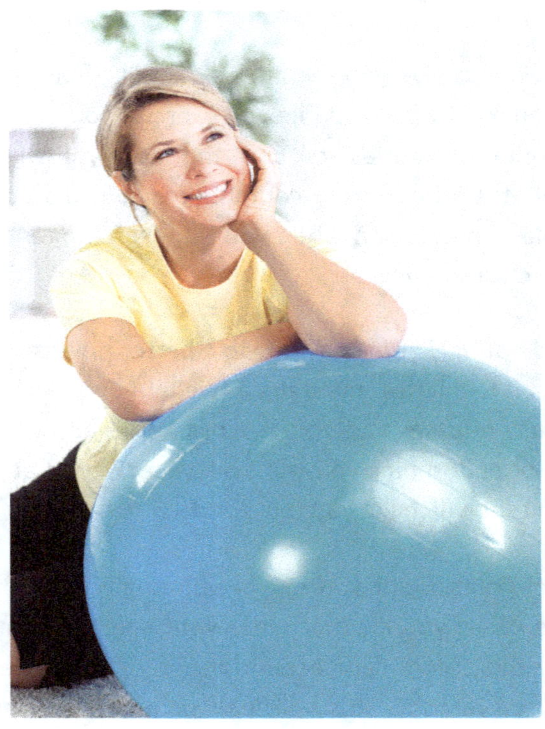

A healthy diet is not the only thing that is important in having a healthier body and mind. It is also important to make sure that you are also getting the right amount of exercise.

At first it may be difficult to get yourself in the routine of exercising on a regular basis. With practice and determination you will find yourself doing it in no time. You will be amazed by how much better you feel every day when you exercise on a regular basis.

Exercise will not only provide you with a healthy body and mind; it will also increase the span of your life. This will give you many extra years to spend with your loved ones.

What Do Babies Eat?

Many people make the error of thinking that a proper diet alone is enough to achieve full body health. This is not the case! A well balanced diet also needs to include regular exercise as this is vital for a person to be healthy.

Exercising will also give you the added benefit of being able to eat more food on a daily basis. While you exercise you burn off fat and calories. The more calories you burn the more you will be able to eat. As well, it will be more acceptable for you to step outside of your diet plan on occasion when you are exercising. After all, you deserve the occasional treat.

Exercise will not only get your body to a better physical state, it will also make you feel better mentally as well. Did you know that your brain naturally releases endorphins while you exercise? When your brain is full of endorphins you will achieve a state of euphoria or a type of high that will make you feel good.

You will feel great about yourself as you begin to see the results from all the effort you have out into your exercise routine. It will make you a more confident person and it will improve your self-worth and self-respect. This will lead to many new great doors opening in your life and ample opportunities. The first thing you need in order to have a happy successful life is a healthy body, spirit, and mind. Exercise can greatly help to improve the state of each one of these.

There is always time to exercise so do not give yourself any excuses. You do not need to do an hour long routine. Doing what you can with the time you have will help. Any effort is still effort.

Richard Parker
What is the Right Exercise Routine for You and Your Lifestyle?

Once you have decided to begin exercising it is important to set up an exercise routine for yourself. This will allow you to make sure that you are getting proper amounts of exercise while exercising different muscle groups and giving you a schedule to stick to.

You need to remember that nobody is going to hold you accountable for bot sticking to that routine but yourself. Slacking off or procrastinating when it comes to your exercise routine will do nothing but slow down the progress of your results which will likely suck your motivation to continue dry.

It is important that you do not try to start your journey to a healthier body and exercise blindly. You need to know some important facts so that you do not injure yourself while trying to better yourself. After all, you do not want to take one step forward and two steps back, do you? I didn't think so. It is always a good idea to consult a trained professional when developing an effective workout routine. These professionals will know the exact routine that will work best with the time you have available, your body type, and the goals that you have in mind.

For those who decide not to use a professional to build their exercise routine, you need to make sure you create a well-balanced exercise routine. You do not want to focus on one muscle group and work on it every day. This can damage muscles over time as they do not have enough time to heal properly. You need to work on different muscle groups on different days of the week. For example, one day you may work on biceps and then the next you work on legs.

If you are exercising for dieting purposes you may want to stick to exercises that focus more on the cardio aspect of things. Treadmills and step climbers can be great ways of burning off carbs and calories. The only problem is the fact that they take up so much space. Most people will not have room in their house for a treadmill so they may have to buy a gym membership. Stationary cycles are also another form of healthy cardio exercises. This type of cardio can be great for older people or those with arthritis as it allows the person working out to sit and take things at their own pace.

There are classes that even incorporate dancing into the cycling to provide an intense workout that is also fun.

If you find yourself having a hard time with sticking to your exercise routine you may want to try adding in some classes that you find fun. The dance exercise craze is exploding and you can find classes for this type of exercise almost anywhere. Programs like Zumba Dance can be quite fun so they hold you attention and bring you back for more and more. During these classes you will have so much fun that you do not even realize you are sweating and burning fat and calories.

Some older individuals may have a hard time bearing weight on their joints. There are special exercise routines that these people can utilize. One example of a form of exercise these older people can still participate in is water aerobics. These water aerobics usually take place in a swimming pool and allow people to exercise without bearing too much weight on their joints. You would be surprised by how well this form of exercise actually works. There is also the option of using workout equipment with counter weights on it. This option is used many times for physical rehabilitation from injuries. It allows the muscles to be strained enough to get exercise but not enough force to damage the persons joints or muscles.

No matter what your exercise goals are, they are accomplishable. All you need to do is find something that you enjoy doing as exercise and before you know it, you will begin to see positive results.

Setting the Right Mindset for Diet and Exercise

The biggest problem that you will face on your journey to a healthier body through diet and exercise will likely be to stay motivated. It can be difficult to continue with your journey at times but it is essential for a better life. Staying motivated is vital if you want to stick to your plans.

One thing that will surely help to keep you motivated is to think of all the hard effort and time you have spent on getting as far as you have with your diet and exercise routine. You do not want to throw it all away do you? Of course not! You need to give yourself credit for the accomplishments you have made so far as well as your progress towards your future goals.

Another good idea is to use your family and friends as a way to keep you motivated. It can be difficult to hold yourself accountable at time because your mind naturally likes to minimize things. Your family and friends can be a good source of honest feedback. Your loved ones and friends will also have a large impact on your thinking if they think that you are starting to lose your motivation. In some cases other people can actually motivate you more than yourself. This is especially true if your health is at risk if you do not continue your diet. Your loved ones should remind you of how much they love you and how much they want you to be healthy. This will make you feel selfish if you start to slack on your diet or exercise and this will likely make you want to get back on track.

What Do Babies Eat?
Some things in this life cannot be accomplished by you on your own and it is ok to reach out for help. Remember, you do not want to go back to square one so catch yourself quickly if you slip so you do not have to climb all the way back up again.

Chapter 8- Don't Let the Diet Plan Do All The Work

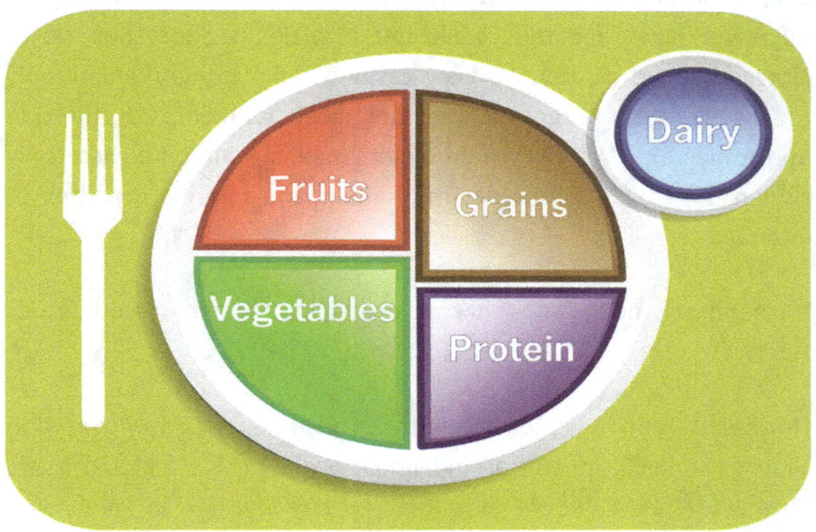

If we hear about the failure of diets or gym plans all around us, commonly it isn't their fault. Commonly it is the fault of the individuals who started with much commotion about going through these plans, telling all their acquaintances and co-workers about it, and then didn't abide by those programs. The individuals who abandon the exercise or diet halfway do not see the advantages, naturally, and everybody blames the plan.

What the world needs nowadays isn't a fresh health or fitness program or a diet, but it requires motivation. It needs the correct sort of mind-set to follow through with whatever plan they have chosen to the very end.

If they can do that, most of the health issues that are related to life-style situations will get to be outmoded. And we don't have to visit the corners of the earth to discover this motivation. The motivation lies right here, inside us; we simply need to search it out and utilize it.

One generation ago, individuals wouldn't dream of picking up whatever junk food they could get in order to feed their faces. Nowadays, we do that so very casually. "I'm hungry" commonly means "I want a burger or a hot dog, likely with chips on the side and some cola." And, "I am on a diet" means "I am on a chemically ridden pill which will defeat my hunger and deprive my body of vitamins."

It's genuinely no wonder that we are facing so many health issues today.

Our health is an indicator of what we consume. The sorry condition that we're living in isn't an individual problem; it's a global issue. The world as a whole is eating incorrectly. Six in every ten individuals in the US is overweight, and the number is going to be eight in every ten individuals by the time we hit 2015.

Are we truly thinking about this? We aren't. Even as you're studying this eBook, you likely have a packet of chips on the side. Do you know that what you spent on that package, which is filling your stomach with some of the most toxic chemicals known to humanity, could instead have fed an emaciated youngster in Ruanda?

But it's not simply about being philanthropic. It's about us too. Yes, we have to be selfish. With such appalling health figures, aren't we heading for doom? We're definitely not eating right. Whatever excess baggage that brings - obesity and the assorted ill health in its wake - we have to be prepared for it.

So the next time you see that a program has failed or is receiving a lot of criticism, remember that the criticism isn't probably because the program stands on shaky ground. In most cases, it is because people began with great intentions and then did not follow the program as they should have.

Your Motivation Keeps Your Diet Plan in Place

Your own motive is the most crucial thing that you need to keep your health and fitness program alive.

You have to be determined to scrutinize the situation. So, you're overweight and are looking at casting off a few pounds. No gym instructor from anyplace in the world will help you if you don't take adequate measures to have the right diet and to stick to your routine exercise.

Even if you're sick and are looking at treatment, no physician will help if you aren't determined in following the treatment platform, whether it's taking the medication at the correct time or abstaining from some foods.

We have strayed horribly with our eating habits thus far. Unless we take stock of the state of affairs and take matters in our own hands, matters are not going to get better.

The number 1 thing is awareness. We have to learn what foods are correct for us and what are not. We have to go back to training and comprehend what the nutrients are that your body truly wants and in what amount.

Then we have to build a dietary regimen for ourselves and our loved ones so that we eat healthier. We have to cut down on all the foods that are adverse - the sugars, the fats, the carbohydrates, we don't truly want them - and incorporate foods that may boost our health.

This does sound too preachy, I understand. But that's the only reprieve we have got. If we continue munching on Oreos, we're never going to get better.

But there's hope. Hope lies in the fact that there are a lot of foods out there that are simply as tasty as those awful junk foods but we don't yet know about them.

These are the foods that we don't know about yet, we likely don't care for them or as we don't know how to fix them, but a healthy cookbook may help you in understanding assorted interesting ways to healthy cooking.

Even with the same sort of diet you eat, you are able to conjure up some really delicious healthy dishes. Yes, it's all very much possible.

You are able to modify your eating habits to a big extent, while at the same time attending to your palate.

The fact is that the weight loss industry is responsible in a really significant way towards this downfall of the developed human race. They have to keep selling their Atkinses and Jenny Craigs and Zones and Medifasts and for that reason the media never tells you how we may in reality take things in your own hands.

They show us glitzy before-after pictures of a person with a foot-long sub and then the same guy with 6 pack abs and tell us that the diet made that possible.

However the fact is if we were to get our head together, we may very easily do that too, without having to spend 1000s of dollars on those diets. And what do we have to do?

2 general things:-

Control what we consume.

Indulge in physical exertion.

Now, is that too much to accomplish? Don't we owe that to our body that has served us so well all these years? Don't we owe that to ourselves and our loved ones?

Track Your Progress

A Really crucial thing for you to do when you're on a health and wellness program is to keep checking how you're progressing. This may keep you highly motivated, particularly when you see that you're becoming what you wish yourself to become.

So, when you're on a diet program, weigh yourself frequently, doesn't matter even if you do it many times a day. When you're jogging, check how many steps you are able to climb without breathing. When you're working out at the gym, monitor the changes in your abs and chest. When you're on a program to better your blood sugar level or your blood pressure, keep monitoring yourself. As a matter of fact, go for more frequent physical checkups just to see how well you're progressing.

Humans are very much result-oriented individuals. We wish to see facts and figures - we wish to see things as raw as they may be. This is the reason why charting your progress continuously may assist you immensely.

What Do Babies Eat?
Once you see that your waist size has come down from 38" to 36", once you see that you are able to get into skimpier shorts, once you see that you're closer to touching your toes than before, you get very much pleased with yourself. You see that your efforts are bearing fruit. This keeps the fire ablaze.

Initially, you'll want to monitor yourself rather often. Your family might even mock you for that. But it doesn't matter. You have to know where you're heading. So keep looking as much as you wish. It is only when you're in love with your body that you'll think of doing something for it. And no one loves your body more than you, so the onus of making it fitter and healthier is totally on you.

You have every right to know how your body is progressing. The best part is that this spurs you on to do better for your body. So keep monitoring yourself and keep working out to your heart's content.

About The Author

Richard Parker is the only son of Dr. Scot Parker and Dr. Mary Lawrence. At an early age, Richard and his family moved to Texas, where his parents built a hospital hoping that someday Richard would run it. But Richard had other plans. He wanted to empower people by being a strong advocate of health and nutrition.

Initially, Richard had a difficult time convincing his parents that he wanted to be a health and nutrition expert, and not a surgeon like them. But when his parents saw how passionate he is in his craft, they started to accept his decision and what was once resistance became support.

Today, Richard owns a gyms and nutrition clubs across Texas.